LIFE SAVING
FOR TEENAGERS

LIFE SAVING

FOR

TEENAGERS

by

C. W. T. COLLIER

M.I.C.E., Dip.R.L.S.S.

DRAKE PUBLISHERS

NEW YORK

ISBN 87749–153–4

Published in 1972 *by*
DRAKE PUBLISHERS INC.
381 *Park Avenue South,*
New York, New York 10016

Library of Congress Catalog Card Number: 75/175790

Printed in Great Britain

CONTENTS

INTRODUCTION

THERE is a large gap between knowing and doing and in an emergency very few people are capable of reacting quickly and correctly without training. Regular practice of the releases, tows and artificial respiration methods is therefore essential to preserve both confidence and a semi-automatic reaction that will overcome the mental panic that can stupefy the mind of even the most intelligent person.

The object of this book is to provide a practical illustrated guide to currently recommended life saving techniques. Action photographs are the principal means used to convey information and the written description has been kept to a minimum.

In addition to the artificial respiration drills, considerable emphasis has been placed on land practices for releases, tows, and where possible, landings. These can be rehearsed in a classroom or gym and give the pupils a better understanding of the movements required, thus enabling them to get the maximum benefit from water practice.

Of course, numerous variations from the basic techniques are possible. The minor variations illustrated require the minimum effort for their execution and are in the author's opinion most suitable for teenagers, though it goes without saying that people of any age will be able to master them without undue difficulty.

INSTRUCTION DRILL FOR
EXPIRED AIR METHOD
OF ARTIFICIAL RESPIRATION

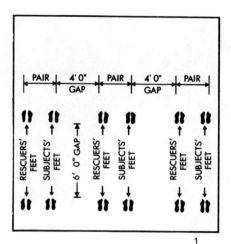

1

"IN PAIRS—FALL IN"

The pairs comprising RESCUER and SUBJECT fall in as shown. RESCUER carries at least two towels.

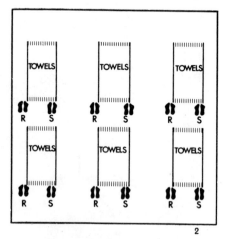

2

"FOR RESUSCITATION WORK—PREPARE"

RESCUERS spread out the towels and return to their original positions.

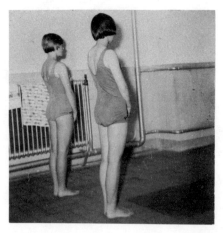

3

NOTE: The verbal commands given are not essential either for instruction or examination purposes. Nevertheless an instructor will find that to control a large group initially, some words of command—not necessarily the ones given—will be useful. At a later stage pupils should be able to practise in pairs without the instructor's supervision.

"FOR RESUSCITATION—CLASS POSITION"

SUBJECT kneels—

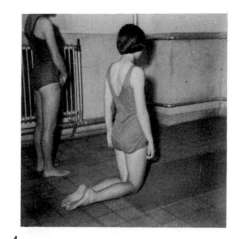

4

—falls forward on her hands—

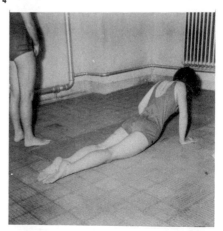

5

—lowers her body onto the mat—

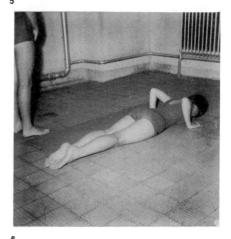

6

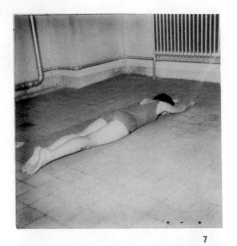

—places her left cheek on the mat and extends both arms above her head.

From this point onwards RESCUER'S movements must be performed with a sense of urgency until the simulated artificial respiration actually begins.

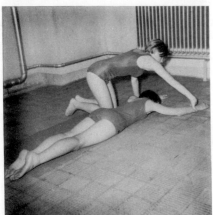

RESCUER moves into the position shown and places SUBJECT'S right hand to her side.

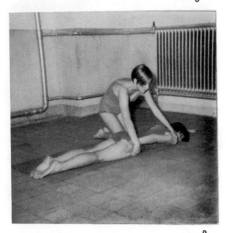

SUBJECT'S right hand is trapped under RESCUER'S right wrist.

12

RESCUER rolls SUBJECT towards
herself by pulling steadily with
both arms. The pull ceases when
SUBJECT is supported by RESCUER'S
thighs.

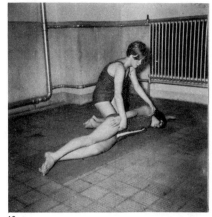

10

RESCUER supports the SUBJECT
on her thighs and inspects her
mouth for possible obstructions such
as seaweed or false teeth. The
inspection is for obvious obstructions
only and consequently should not
require more than two seconds.

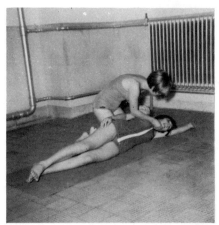

11

RESCUER'S hands now change
position to support SUBJECT'S head
with the left hand and SUBJECT'S
shoulder with the left forearm.
RESCUER'S right hand slides beneath
SUBJECT'S hip.

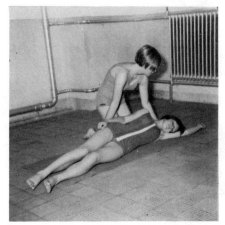

12

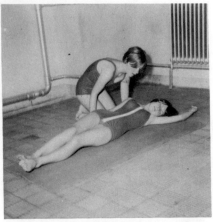

RESCUER adjusts her kneeling position and eases SUBJECT onto her back.

13

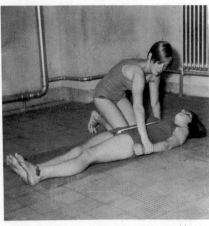

RESCUER moves SUBJECT's left arm to her side.

Having observed that SUBJECT's face, ears, lips and fingernail beds are purple, RESCUER decides that artificial respiration will be necessary.

14

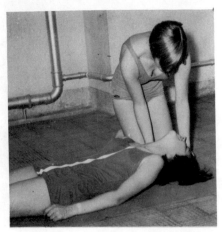

RESCUER moves on her knees to a position near to the SUBJECT's head and extends her neck by lifting with the right hand under the neck and pushing the top of the head downwards with the left hand.

The neck extension is very important. It ensures that an unconscious SUBJECT's tongue is moved away from the back of her throat, thus providing a clear air passage to the lungs.

15

RESCUER's thumb is on the chin, her index and middle fingers under the jawbone, the other fingers curled into her palm. RESCUER is about to demonstrate the mouth-to-nose method and consequently pushes SUBJECT's jaw towards the top of her head to ensure that the mouth remains closed. RESCUER's left hand maintains a constant downward pressure on the top of SUBJECT's head to keep her neck extended.

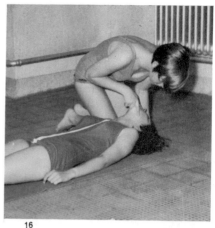

16

"RESUSCITATION—COM-MENCE"

RESCUER's face is positioned at least six inches above SUBJECT's face and just beyond her left cheek. RESCUER *does NOT breathe into* SUBJECT's *nose*. The first four breaths "are deep and rapid", after which a rate of twelve to fifteen times a minute is maintained. RESCUER maintains the required rate by counting mentally "one and two and three" as she exhales steadily and audibly.

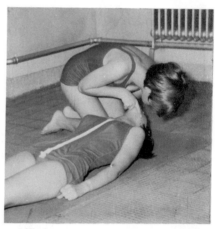

17

RESCUER turns her head ostensibly to watch SUBJECT's chest fall—and inhales deeply to a mental count of "four and five and six" in readiness to exhale as shown above. RESCUER continues the expiration and inspiration for approximately one minute.

A stop watch placed on the mat below RESCUER's face provides an excellent check on the rate of breathing.

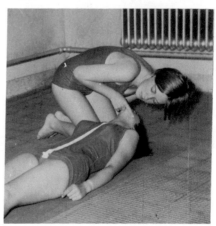

18

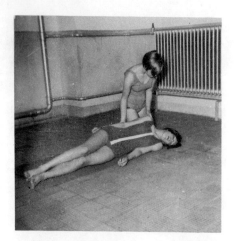

19

"CLASS HALT. ON TO THE SIDE—TURN."

RESCUER raises SUBJECT'S right shoulder and supports her back on the right thigh. This action must be performed quickly to obviate the possibility of SUBJECT being further asphyxiated with her own vomit.

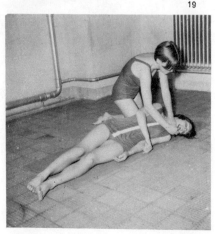

20

RESCUER goes through the motions of clearing SUBJECT'S mouth of vomit.

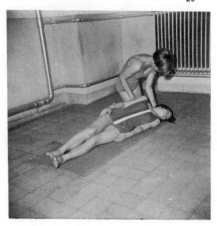

21

"RESUME POSITION."

RESCUER lowers SUBJECT onto her back, supporting the right shoulder with her right hand whilst she repositions her right knee. RESCUER'S left hand supports SUBJECT'S head.

"RESUSCITATION—COMMENCE."

The movements described opposite photographs 17 and 18 are repeated but simulating the mouth to-mouth technique as demonstrated in photograph 27.

16

"RESUSCITATION HALT."

RESCUER ceases the breathing movements and stands to attention near SUBJECT'S right hip.

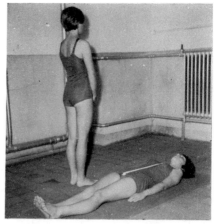

22

"REFORM."

SUBJECT bends her right leg and raises her right arm. RESCUER grasps SUBJECT'S right hand in both her own and assists her to rise.

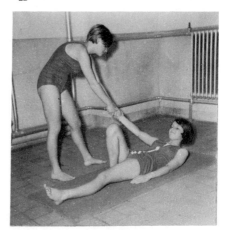

23

"PLACES—CHANGE."

RESCUER now moves to the right and SUBJECT to the left to take up the positions shown.

The entire drill is then repeated using the same orders.

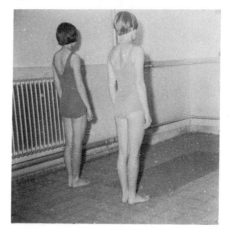

24

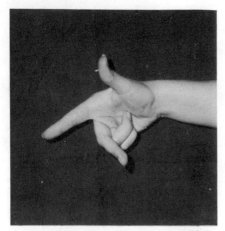

25

HAND POSITION.

The index and middle fingers are placed on either side and underneath SUBJECT's jawbone, thumb on the chin and the remaining two fingers curled into the palm to keep them away from SUBJECT's throat.

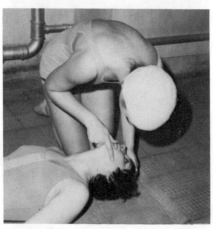

26

MOUTH-TO-NOSE.

RESCUER is pushing SUBJECT's jawbone upwards with the index and middle fingers to keep the mouth closed. The thumb is on the chin but remains passive.

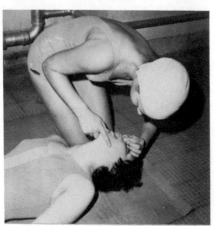

27

MOUTH-TO-MOUTH.

RESCUER has opened SUBJECT's mouth by pressing down with the thumb on SUBJECT's chin. The index and middle fingers do not apply any pressure. The heel of RESCUER's other hand is pressed down on SUBJECT's forehead to maintain the necessary neck extension while the fingers close the nose.

ALTERNATIVE HAND POSITION.

The thumb and index fingers are placed on either side of the jawbone and the other fingers curled into the palm of the hand.

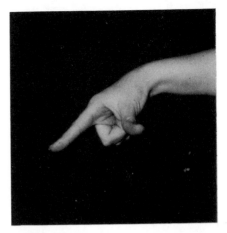

28

MOUTH-TO-NOSE.

RESCUER is pushing SUBJECT'S jawbone upwards with the curled middle finger to keep the mouth closed. The thumb and index finger remain passive.

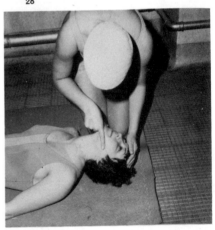

29

MOUTH-TO-MOUTH.

RESCUER has opened SUBJECT'S mouth by pulling her jawbone downwards with the thumb and index finger. The curled middle finger does not exert any pressure. The heel of RESCUER'S other hand is pressed down on SUBJECT'S forehead to maintain the necessary neck extension while the fingers close the nose.

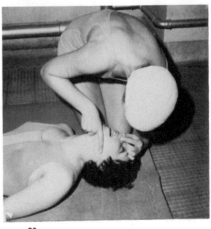

30

INSTRUCTION DRILL FOR
SILVESTER-BROSCH METHOD
OF ARTIFICIAL RESPIRATION

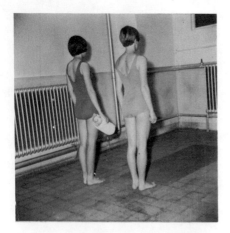

"FOR RESUSCITATION WORK—PREPARE."

RESCUER folds at least two thick towels once lengthwise and then rolls them tightly.

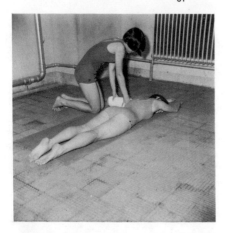

31

"FOR RESUSCITATION CLASS—POSITION."

The actions shown in photographs 1 to 7 are repeated.

RESCUER moves into position shown and places the rolled towels immediately opposite SUBJECT'S shoulder blades.

32

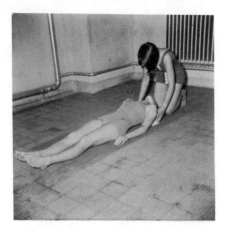

The actions shown in photographs 8 to 14 are repeated.

RESCUER moves around to SUBJECT'S head and adjusts the rolled towels as necessary to make certain that the back of SUBJECT'S head is barely touching the ground, thus ensuring a good neck extension.

33

RESCUER adopts the position
shown, with the toes of her left foot
placed immediately below SUBJECT'S
left shoulder. RESCUER'S right knee
is just clear of the top of SUBJECT'S
head and the inside of the right
thigh in line with SUBJECT'S right ear.

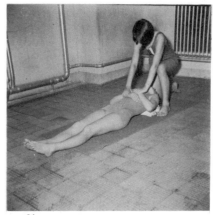

34

"RESUSCITATION—COM-
MENCE."

RESCUER with arms straight,
rocks forward gently until they are
vertical and applying pressure to the
sternum to a mental count of "one
and two" (the force applied should be
22 to 30 lb. for adults, 12 to 14 lb.
for slight women and children and
2 to 4 lb. for infants).

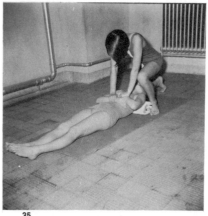

35

RESCUER rocks back releasing
the pressure and lifting SUBJECT'S
arms. The mental count continues
'and".

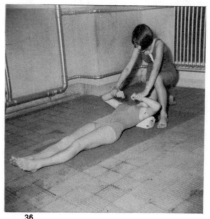

36

23

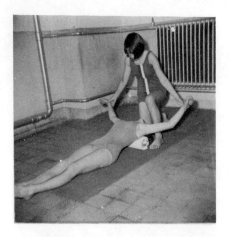

RESCUER continues moving SUBJECT'S arms outwards in a semi-circular sweep. The mental count continues "three".

37

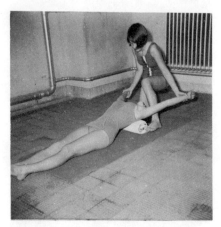

The sweep is continued until SUBJECT'S arms are extended above her head. RESCUER must *not* force SUBJECT'S arms to the ground in this position. The mental count continues "and four".

The time taken in lifting SUBJECT'S arms from her chest into the extended position shown is two seconds.

The full extension of SUBJECT'S arms should produce a clearly visible expansion of her rib cage.

38

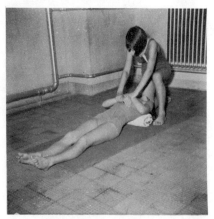

SUBJECT'S arms are returned to their original position on SUBJECT'S chest with a similar semi-circular sweep. The mental count continues "and five and six". Returning SUBJECT'S arms to her chest occupies two seconds.

The complete cycle of movements requires five seconds and is performed continuously for one minute. Practice this with a stop watch.

39

"CLASS—HALT. ONTO THE SIDE—TURN."

RESCUER moves around to the side of SUBJECT's head and raises her right shoulder. RESCUER then supports SUBJECT's back on her right thigh.

After a short pause to enable the SUBJECT to finish vomiting, the motions of clearing the SUBJECT's mouth shown in photograph 20 are repeated.

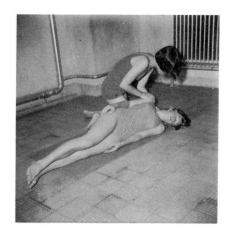

40

"RESUME POSITION".

The actions described opposite photograph 21 are repeated.

RESCUER then adjusts the rolled towels as shown.

"RESUSCITATION—COMMENCE."

The movements described opposite photographs 34 to 39 inclusive, are repeated for a further one minute.

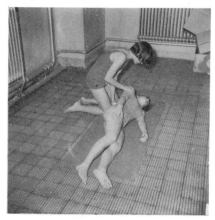

41

"CLASS—HALT."

RESCUER completes the five second cycle by returning SUBJECT's arms to her chest and stands up at attention near SUBJECT's right hip.

"RE-FORM."

The actions described opposite photograph 23 are repeated.

"PLACES—CHANGE."

As for photograph 24.

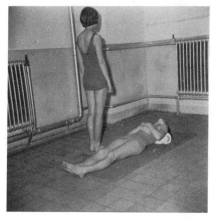

25   42

INSTRUCTION DRILL FOR
EXTERNAL CARDIAC COMPRESSION

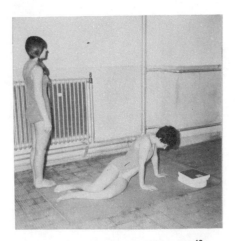

43

"FOR RESUSCITATION, CLASS—POSITION."

The SUBJECT kneels as illustrated in photograph 4, and turns as shown.

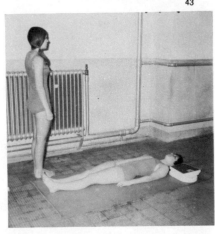

44

SUBJECT lies face upwards with her arms to her sides.

From this point onwards RESCUER'S movements must be performed with a sense of urgency until the simulated artificial respiration begins.

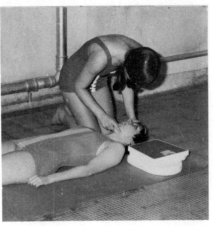

45

RESCUER moves forward to SUBJECT'S head and inspects her mouth for possible obstructions. The obstructions will be obvious ones, such as seaweed or false teeth and consequently the inspection should not require more than two seconds.

RESCUER extends SUBJECT'S neck
and performs actions described
and shown in photographs 15 and 16.
RESCUER breathes deeply while performing these actions to build up
the oxygen content in her lungs.

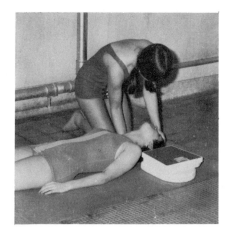

46

"RESUSCITATION—COM-
MENCE."
   RESCUER carries out actions
shown in photographs 17 and 18 for
four rapid cycles.

   RESCUER then examines SUBJECT'S
pupils.

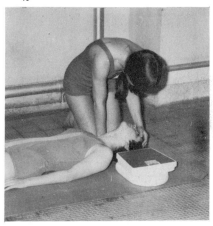

47

   RESCUER feels for the carotid
pulse and checks SUBJECT'S colour.

   Having found that:
(a) SUBJECT'S pupils are dilated.
(b) SUBJECT has no carotid pulse.
(c) SUBJECT'S face is a blue-grey
     colour.
RESCUER decides that external cardiac
compression is necessary.

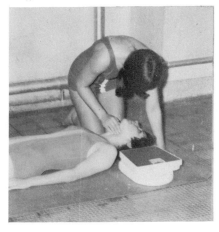

48

29

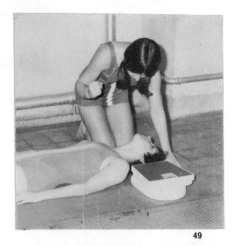

RESCUER goes through the motions of striking the SUBJECT'S sternum with a clenched fist.

This action is *not* repeated again during the continuation of the drill.

49

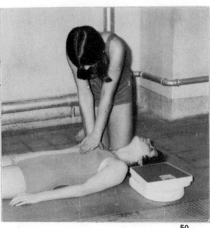

RESCUER checks carotid pulse again as in photograph 48 to ascertain if striking the sternum has been sufficient to start the heart beating.

Failing to feel any pulse RESCUER places the heel of one hand on SUBJECT'S sternum, the other hand is placed on top. This position is held for a few seconds but *no pressure is actually applied.*

50

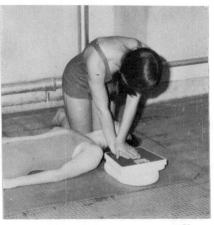

RESCUER repositions her hands onto the bathroom scale and applies a force of 4 to 5 stones at the rate of one compression per second by swinging her body backwards and forwards. After five to eight compressions RESCUER extends SUBJECT'S neck and repeats one cycle of the Expired Air Method as illustrated in photographs 15 to 18.

The entire drill is repeated until the command "Resuscitation—Halt" is given—see photograph 22. "Reform"—see photograph 23. "Places Change"—see photograph 24

51

30

COMPRESSION.

The hands are placed one on top of the other with fingers of both hands parallel thus ensuring straight arms for the efficient transmission of RESCUER's body weight onto SUBJECT's sternum. The fingers of both hands are raised slightly to concentrate the pressure area under the heel of one hand when RESCUER rocks forward.

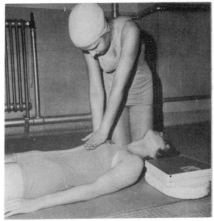

52

CHECKING THE PULSE.

RESCUER has placed her fingers just under and along SUBJECT's sterno-mastoid muscle to feel her carotid pulse.

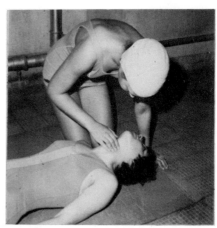

53

COMA POSITION.

SUBJECT is breathing but unconscious. This position prevents the unconscious SUBJECT's tongue from blocking the airway.

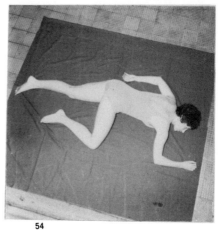

54

31

LAND PRACTICE FOR RELEASES

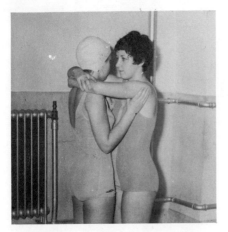

55

FRONT CLUTCH ROUND NECK.

RESCUER may be clutched round the neck in any of the following grip variations.

If clutched very closely, RESCUER immediately prepares to break the clutch by dropping her chin, contracting the neck muscles and placing her hands under SUBJECT'S armpits. RESCUER is now ready to perform the Push Away Break.

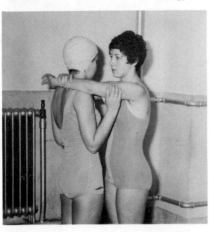

56

If clutched as shown, RESCUER can prepare to make the release by placing her hands on SUBJECT'S upper arms.

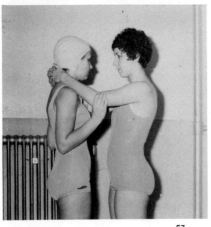

57

If clutched round the neck with SUBJECT'S forearms bearing down on RESCUER'S chest, RESCUER places her hands under SUBJECT'S elbows.

RELEASE FROM FRONT CLUTCH ROUND NECK—
using Push Away Break.

SUBJECT grips RESCUER around the neck with forearms bearing on her chest.

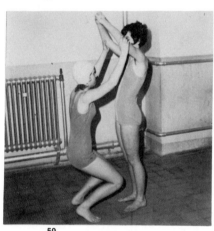

58

RESCUER places her hands under SUBJECT'S elbows, tucks her chin well in, takes a deep breath then jerks SUBJECT'S elbows upwards and submerges.

59

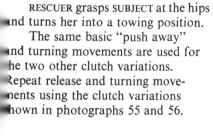

RESCUER grasps SUBJECT at the hips and turns her into a towing position.

The same basic "push away" and turning movements are used for the two other clutch variations. Repeat release and turning movements using the clutch variations shown in photographs 55 and 56.

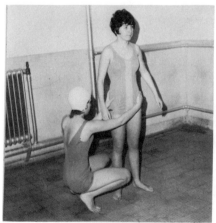

60

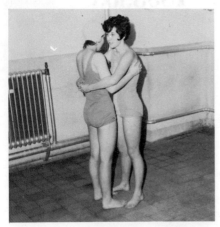

RELEASE FROM FRONT CLUTCH ROUND BODY—
using Push Away Break.

SUBJECT grasps RESCUER around the body pinning her arms to her sides. RESCUER places both her hands under SUBJECT's armpits.

61

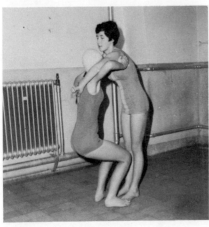

RESCUER takes a deep breath, tucks her chin into her shoulder and submerges by forcing her elbows outwards and upwards.

62

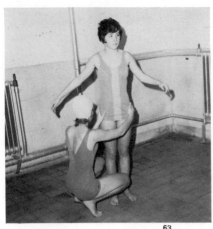

While in the submerged position RESCUER turns SUBJECT ready for towing by gripping SUBJECT's hips with both hands, pulling with one and pushing with the other.

63

RELEASE FROM WRIST GRIP—
using Pull Control.

SUBJECT grips RESCUER's wrist
with both hands.

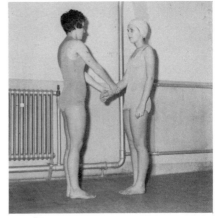

64

RESCUER has pulled SUBJECT
towards herself and is throwing her
free arm around SUBJECT's neck
as she passes.

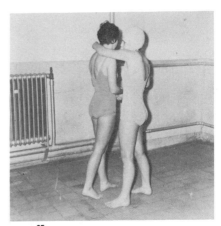

65

RESCUER is bearing down on SUBJECT's
shoulder with the forearm of the
hand gripping the chin.

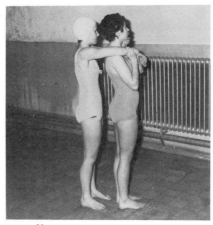

66

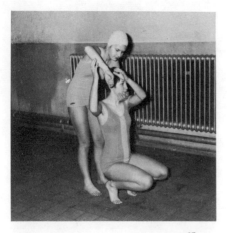

SUBJECT has been forced down
and RESCUER is freeing her arm.

67

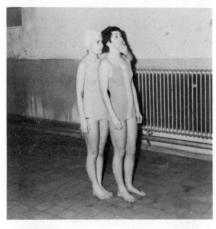

RESCUER has raised SUBJECT by
the chin onto her shoulder in
readiness for the Chin Tow.

68

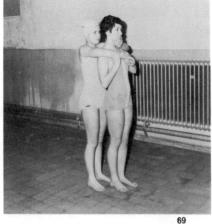

If RESCUER fails to free her
clutched wrist she allows it to remain
held by the SUBJECT for the remainder of the tow.

Repeat the release with SUBJECT
gripping the other wrist.

69

RELEASE FROM WRIST GRIP—
using Arm Pull Up.

RESCUER'S wrist has been gripped by SUBJECT with her thumbs on top. RESCUER has clenched the fist of the gripped wrist and grasped it with her free hand.

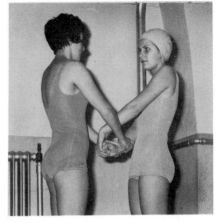

70

RESCUER is pulling her own fist upwards against SUBJECT'S thumbs and SUBJECT is releasing her grip.

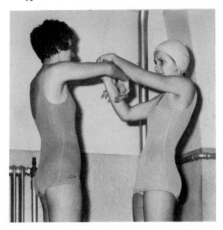

71

RESCUER is turning SUBJECT. Repeat the release with SUBJECT gripping the other wrist.

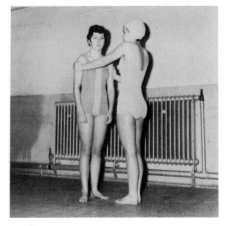

72

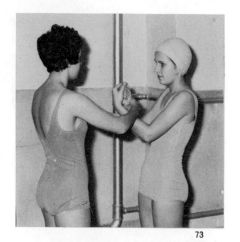

73

RELEASE FROM WRIST GRIP— using Arm Pull Down.

RESCUER'S wrist has been gripped by SUBJECT with her thumbs underneath. RESCUER has clenched the fist of the gripped wrist and grasped it with her free hand.

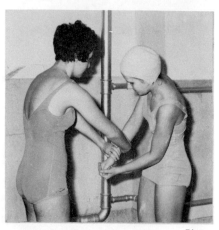

74

RESCUER is pulling her own fist downwards against SUBJECT'S thumbs to break the grip.

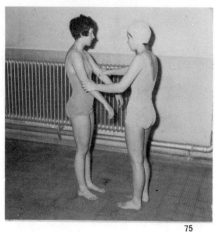

75

RESCUER has grasped SUBJECT at the elbows ready to turn her into a towing position by pushing with one arm and pulling with the other.

Repeat the movements with SUBJECT gripping the other wrist.

RELEASE FROM BACK CLUTCH ROUND NECK—
using Elbow Break

RESCUER grips SUBJECT'S uppermost wrist with one hand, thumb on top, while RESCUER'S other hand grips SUBJECT'S elbow. RESCUER turns her head away from SUBJECT'S gripped elbow.

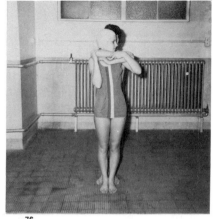

76

RESCUER pushes SUBJECT'S elbow up and pulls her wrist down to pass under the gripped arm.

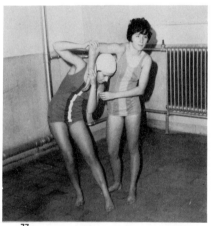

77

RESCUER carries SUBJECT'S arm around behind her back.

Repeat practice with SUBJECT'S left arm uppermost.

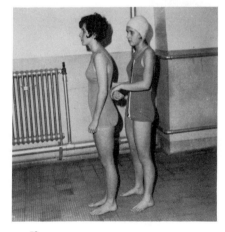

78

41

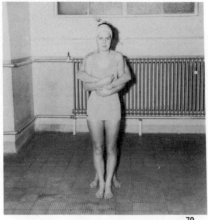

RELEASE FROM BACK CLUTCH ROUND BODY—
using Joint Pressure Break.

RESCUER grips SUBJECT'S thumb with one hand and fingers with the other hand in readiness to force SUBJECT'S hands apart by applying pressure, principally against the thumb joint.

79

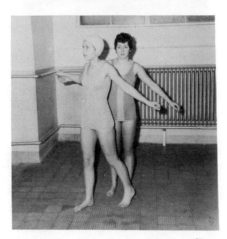

Having broken the hold, RESCUER spreads SUBJECT'S arms wide to escape.

80

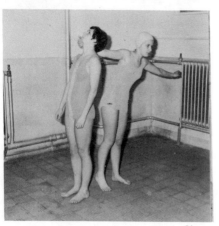

RESCUER has moved around behind SUBJECT and taken hold of her chin ready for towing.

81

42

SEPARATION OF TWO SWIMMERS LOCKED TOGETHER— with a body grip.

RESCUER approaches the weaker SUBJECT (hands around other SUBJECT'S body) from behind and grips her chin with both hands, fingers interlaced. RESCUER bears down with her forearms on the weaker SUBJECT'S shoulders to sink both SUBJECTS.

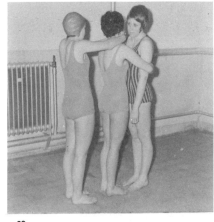

82

RESCUER places her foot on the gripped SUBJECT'S shoulder opposite to the one on which the weaker SUBJECT'S head lies.

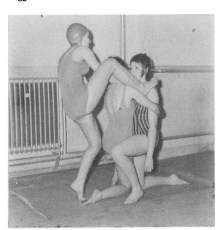

83

RESCUER breaks the hold by pushing with her leg and pulling upwards and backwards with her hands.

N.B. For the first few land practices, the presence of a "catcher" positioned immediately behind RESCUER, is recommended in case she overbalances.

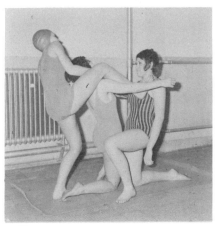

84

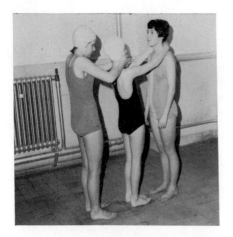

SEPARATION OF TWO SWIMMERS LOCKED TOGETHER—
with a neck grip.

RESCUER approaches the weaker swimmer from behind and grips her chin with both hands, fingers interlaced. RESCUER bears down with her forearms on the weaker swimmer's shoulders to sink both SUBJECTS.

85

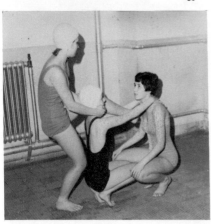

Having submerged both SUBJECTS, RESCUER brings her foot over the weaker SUBJECT'S shoulder and places it on the other SUBJECT'S chest.

86

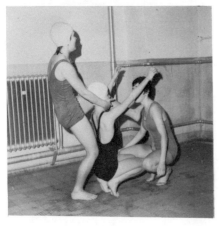

RESCUER breaks the hold by pushing with her leg and pulling upwards and backwards with her hands.

N.B. The assistance of two "catchers", one behind SUBJECT, the other behind RESCUER is recommended.

87

LAND PRACTICE FOR
TOWING METHODS

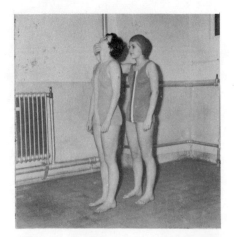

CHIN TOW—

used to tow a passive subject and easily adapted to retrain one who struggles. RESCUER uses the life saving backstroke kick throughout all the restraints when in the water.

RESCUER has passed her hand over SUBJECT'S shoulder to grip her chin.

88

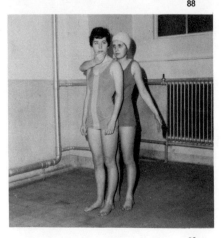

Towing method for a passive subject.

Points of technique:
(1) RESCUER turns SUBJECT'S face towards her own.
(2) RESCUER keeps as much as possible of her forearm pressed against SUBJECT'S chest.
(3) RESCUER uses her free hand to assist the tow by sculling.

89

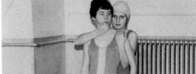

SHOULDER RESTRAINT.

If SUBJECT struggles, RESCUER passes her free hand under SUBJECT'S armpit and grips her shoulder.

90

BREATHING RESTRAINT.

If SUBJECT persists in struggling RESCUER grips SUBJECT'S nose between her thumb and forefinger at the same time covering the mouth with her hand.

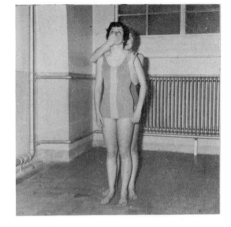

91

SUBJECT instinctively grabs RESCUER'S arm to pull the hand away from the face.

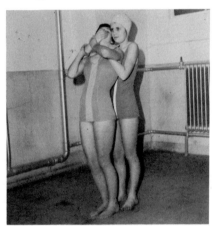

92

SUBJECT has pulled RESCUER'S arm down onto her chest. RESCUER has removed her hand from SUBJECT'S shoulder and is now able to use it again to assist the tow by sculling. The position shown may be maintained until the completion of the tow.

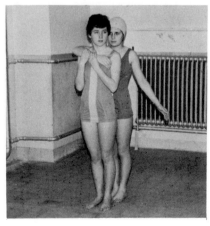

93

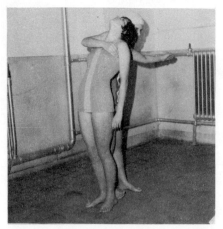

CROSS CHEST TOW—
to tow a passive SUBJECT—using the side stroke kick.

Points of technique:
(1) RESCUER holds SUBJECT firmly against her side.
(2) RESCUER keeps her hip close to the small of SUBJECT's back.
(3) The arm holding SUBJECT should be bent to about a right angle to avoid the possibility of RESCUER's forearm pressing against SUBJECT's throat.

94

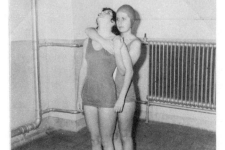

CROSS CHEST TOW—
with restraint—to tow a struggling SUBJECT using the backstroke kick.

RESCUER has passed her hand underneath SUBJECT's armpit to grip her shoulder. RESCUER uses the life saving backstroke kick for the duration of the restraint only.

95

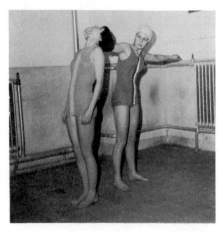

EXTENDED TOW—
to tow a passive SUBJECT—using the side stroke kick.

Points of technique:
(1) Hold SUBJECT's chin firmly with fingers away from her throat.
(2) RESCUER flexes her arm and wrist as necessary to keep SUBJECT's mouth and nose clear of the water.
(3) RESCUER holds SUBJECT's head over her hip when towing.

96

DOUBLE RESCUE TOW—
by the chin with extended arms—to tow two passive SUBJECTS using the life saving backstroke kick.

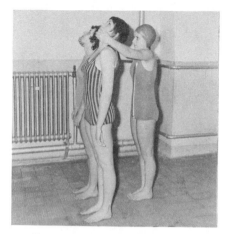

97

DOUBLE RESCUE TOW—
by the chin with bent arms.

This is a personal variation preferred by RESCUER.

Points of technique:
(1) Grip SUBJECTS' chins firmly.
(2) Keep the little finger edge of the hands away from SUBJECTS' throats.
(3) Keep SUBJECTS apart—if SUBJECTS' shoulders touch during the tow it upsets their balance.

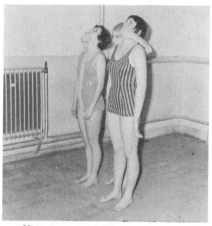

98

DOUBLE RESCUE TOW—
by the hair with extended arms.

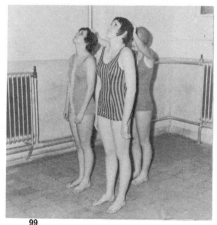

99

49

PRELIMINARY PRACTICE
FOR LANDINGS

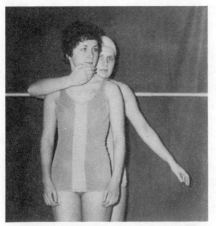

100

LANDING A RESCUED SUBJECT
—preliminary movements only.

SUBJECT has been brought to the bank using the Chin Tow.

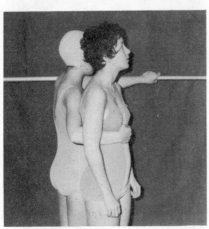

101

RESCUER grasps the bar, then quickly moves her other hand from the chin to just below SUBJECT'S sternum. SUBJECT is held firmly against RESCUER'S right front side and turned to face the bar.

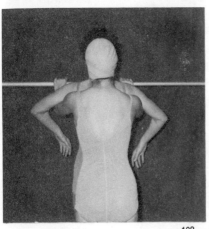

102

RESCUER has grasped the bar with her right hand then released her grip with the left hand to pass it under SUBJECT'S left arm and grip the bar to obtain the "support" position.

52

While retaining a firm grip on the bar with her left hand RESCUER grasps SUBJECT'S right wrist over-hand and places it on the wall (which represents the bank).

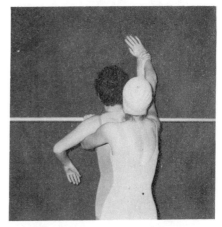

103

RESCUER, supporting all her weight on her right hand releases the bar with her left hand and grasps SUBJECTS left hand to place it on top of SUBJECT'S right hand.

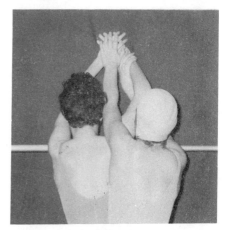

104

RESCUER withdraws her right hand, leaving both SUBJECT'S hands covered by the left hand. RESCUER, supporting as much weight as possible on her left hand, moves to SUBJECT'S right and places her free right hand on the wall (representing the bank).

The complete landing using the Crossed Arm Method and the Straight Arm Method is illustrated later on pages 96-99.

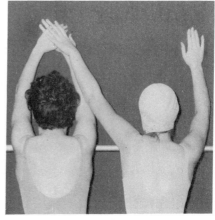

105

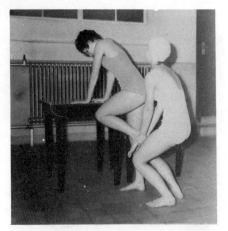

106

LANDING A CO-OPERATIVE SUBJECT—
using the Stirrup Method.

RESCUER instructs SUBJECT to "place both hands on the table and raise your left foot". SUBJECT, standing with her right hip near the table, carries out the instructions. RESCUER keeping her back as vertical as possible, bends her knees and grips SUBJECT's foot firmly with both hands, fingers interlaced.

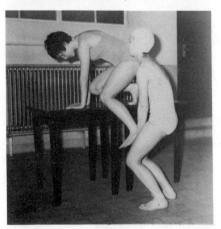

107

RESCUER instructs SUBJECT to "straighten your leg and push up with your arms". RESCUER straightens her knees, while keeping her back as upright as possible, to lift SUBJECT's foot.

SUBJECT can assist the lift considerably by a spring from the foot on which she is standing.

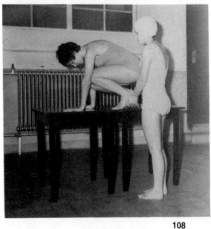

108

Having completely straightened her legs, RESCUER follows through by bending her arms to finally lift and place SUBJECT's foot on the table.

PERSONAL SKILLS

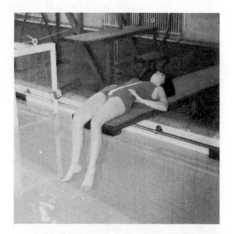

LIFE SAVING BACKSTROKE KICK—

land demonstration of preliminary practice movements.

Recovery

After completion of the glide RESCUER'S knees are bent until the position illustrated is achieved.

109

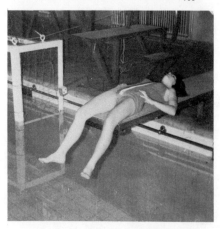

Propulsion

The lower legs now make a circular motion outwards and up-wards with the feet splayed so that the insides of the feet and legs push the water.

110

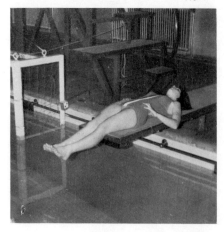

Glide

The propulsive movement is completed by bringing the legs together near the surface of the water in the glide position as shown.

111

LIFE SAVING BACKSTROKE KICK—

preliminary water practice of basic movements.

Recovery

The knees are bent, the body almost horizontal, the top of the thighs are in line with the front of the body and just below the surface of the water.

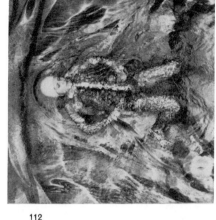

112

Propulsion

The feet are splayed out so that the insides of the feet and legs push the water in a circular motion outwards and upwards.

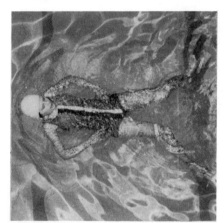

113

Glide

The extended legs have come together in line with the body.

When towing a SUBJECT the glide is practically non-existent, the legs only being extended for the briefest instant before the lower legs again descend to produce another propulsive movement.

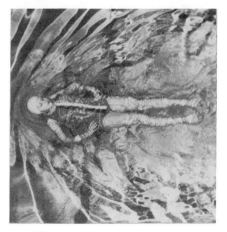

114

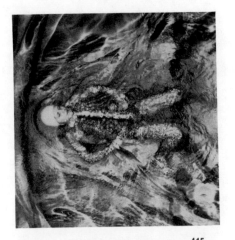

LIFE SAVING BACKSTROKE
KICK—training.

While learning the stroke the
hands are placed on the hips,
the arms projecting outwards below
the water on each side thus improving
the pupil's lateral stability. The
glide is now omitted and the feet
make continuous circular movements
to produce steady progress without
jerking.

115

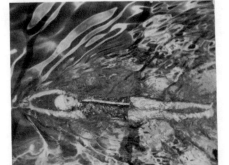

Arms are extended above the
head with the thumbs locked. This is
a useful position for correcting
"sitters" (i.e. pupils who bend at the
hips when performing the stroke).

116

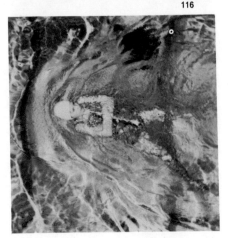

Arms are folded on the chest.
Parts of the pupil's arms will be
above the water causing her to sink
slightly thus producing conditions
a little nearer to actual towing.
The feet make continuous circular
movements. This is the best training
position in which to improve power,
speed and distance.

117

SIDE STROKE—land demonstration.

Recovery
On completion of the glide
RESCUER'S legs part (as in walking)
and the knees are bent. The hand of
the uppermost arm is just below
the face with the elbow close to the
body. The other arm has just
completed a shallow pull from a
fully extended position back to the
shoulder.

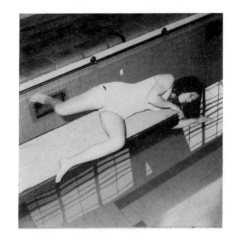

118

Propulsion
The legs are scissored together
with the legs straight and the ankles
extended. The lowest arm is extended
forward with the palm downwards
as the uppermost arm makes a
shallow pull backwards.

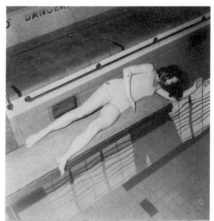

119

Glide
The legs are together with
ankles extended. The lower arm is
fully stretched forwards while the
upper arm, having completed its
backward pull is lying alongside the
thigh.

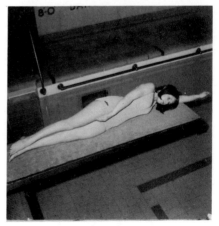

120

SIDE STROKE—in the water.

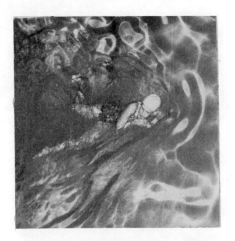

121

Recovery

Pupil's recovery has been made in preparation for the inverted scissor kick, i.e. the lower leg (in this illustration the left) is forward. Most pupils prefer to use the orthodox kick with the upper leg forward on recovery and lie on their right side. Inhale as lower arm pulls down.

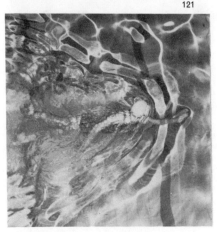

122

Propulsion

Both legs must close horizontally. Exhale.

[When attempting this stroke initially many pupils produce a modified breast stroke kick which must be avoided.]

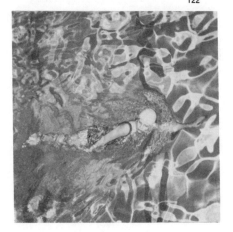

123

Glide

Hold this position for a short interval. As soon as speed begins to fall another stroke is commenced. Exhalation completed.

SURFACE DIVE—head first.

Approach
  RESCUER approaches the block
swimming breast stroke. As soon as
the legs have closed for the glide
position the body is bent at the hips
—by pulling down vigorously with
the arms and depressing the head—
until the upper part of the trunk
is pointing downwards.

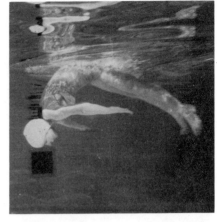

124

Dive
  The legs, straight and together,
are raised quickly into the air,
bringing the whole body back into
line. RESCUER's palms are turned
outwards ready for a breast stroke
arm action to achieve greater depth
rapidly.

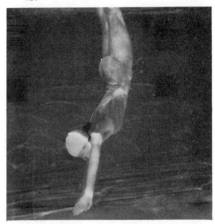

125

Grasping Block
  Near the bottom of the bath the
head is raised to look at the block,
thus arching the back and causing
RESCUER's surface dive to flatten out.
The block is grasped with both
hands.
  [The block, between 5 and 10
lbs. in weight, represents the head of
an unconscious SUBJECT.]

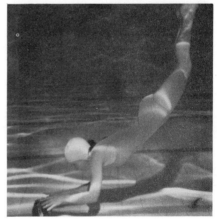

126

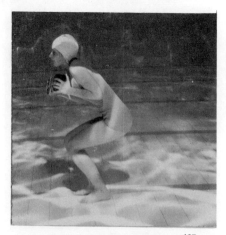

Preparation for Push-off
The block is held firmly with both hands against the chest and just below the chin. The legs are bent ready to push vigorously.

127

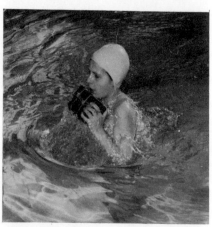

Surfacing
From a depth of seven feet, the head and chest should rise clear above the surface of the water as a result of the push-off.

128

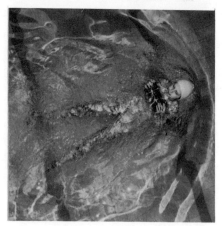

Return to Bank
RESCUER, using the life saving back stroke kick, swims with the block to the bath side. Grasping the rail with one hand, she uses the other hand to place the block on the bank.

129

SURFACE DIVE—feet first.

RESCUER approaching the block swimming breast stroke, stops and treads water above the block.

Push-up

RESCUER, with her body in an upright position gives a strong breast stroke kick simultaneously pressing downwards with both hands from the surface of the water to raise her body as high as possible out of the water.

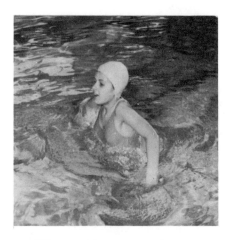

130

Dive

RESCUER taking a deep breath, raises her arms above her head. Toes are pointed and her legs together.

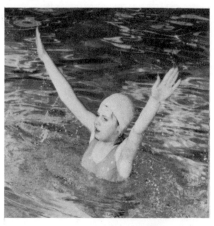

131

Grasping Block

RESCUER'S feet are placed near the block, and the knees partly bent as the block is grasped.

The return to the surface and the bank are as illustrated for the head first surface dive. [Photographs 27, 128 and 129.]

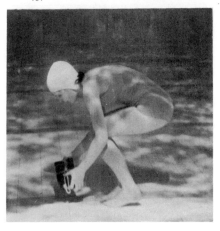

132

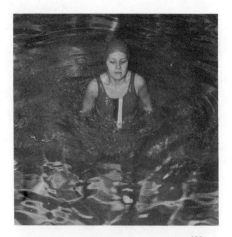

SURFACE DIVE—
feet first—alternative method.

From an upright position approximately above the block RESCUER gives a powerful upward breastroke kick and simultaneously pushes the water downwards from the surface with both hands until they reach her sides.

133

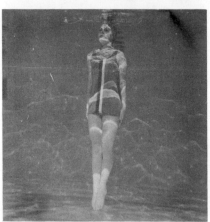

RESCUER'S hands remain at her sides until the top of her head is below the surface of the water. RESCUER points her toes to reduce the resistance to her descent.

134

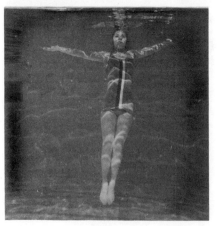

As soon as RESCUER'S head is below the surface, the arms, palms uppermost sweep upwards to thrust her farther down towards the block. [Photographs 132, 127, 128 and 129 illustrate the continuation of this technique.]

135

SCULLING—hand movements.

Sculling is essentially a hand movement, the forearm muscles providing the main propulsive power. The arms remain straight and fairly close to the sides.

The photograph on the left illustrates the head first technique pushing the water towards the feet. The adjacent photograph shows the water being pushed towards the head.

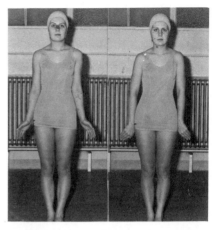

136

SCULLING—head first.

The body is practically horizontal with the head tilted forward slightly to look at the pointed toes which remain just above the surface of the water. The hands perform continuous circular movements with emphasis on the action of pushing the water towards the feet.

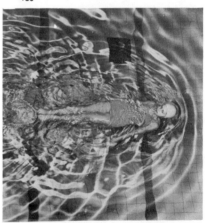

137

SCULLING—feet first.

Adopt the same position as before. The circular hand movements now push the water towards the head.

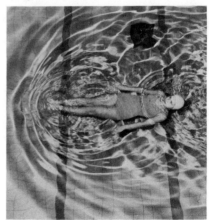

138

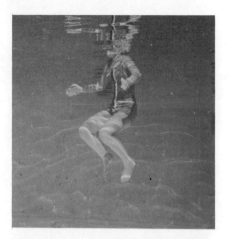

TREADING WATER—
using arms and legs.

The legs perform a breast stroke kick while the hands make any sculling or waving action that thrusts the water downwards. The head is tilted back to immerse the back of the head and keep the mouth and nose clear of the water.

139

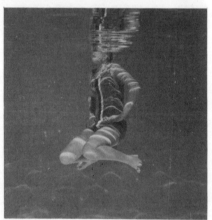

TREADING WATER—
using legs only.

Hands are placed on hips while legs perform a breast stroke kick.

140

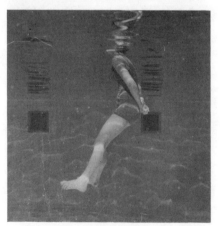

TREADING WATER—
using legs only.

Hands are clasped behind the back while legs perform a breast stroke kick.

141

VERTICAL FLOATING—
arms only.

Hands make any movements that thrust the water downwards, legs are held together and head tilted back.

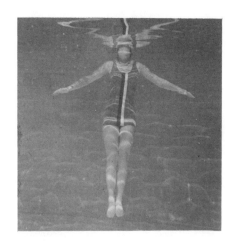

142

VERTICAL FLOATING—
without using arms or legs.

Arms are held to the sides and legs together. The head is held well back so that as much of the head as practicable is below the surface. Breathing is shallow to retain as much air as possible in the lungs.

N.B. This technique is not included in R.L.S.S. syllabus of skills.

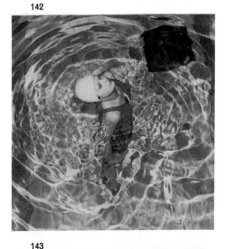

143

Vertical floating position, without using arms or legs, viewed from below.

As an alternative to shallow breathing, "explosive breathing" (a rapid, forceful exhalation followed immediately by a quick inhalation through the mouth) may be used.

This is an excellent exercise for improving self confidence and control.

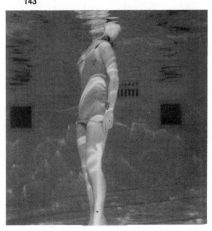

67   144

SHALLOW DIVE—
from the bath side.

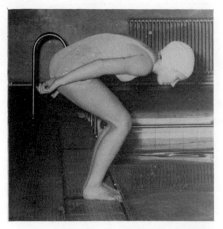

RESCUER'S toes are curled over the bath edge and her knees bent. The arms have just reached their maximum backward movement before swinging vigorously forward for entry.

145

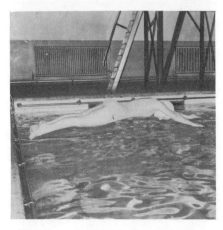

RESCUER'S arms have swung forward as her legs straightened to give the maximum forward drive. The head is well down with the upper arms touching the ears.

146

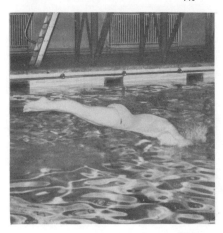

RESCUER'S entry angle is shallow in order to achieve the maximum distance and she will not submerge more than about two feet below the surface of the water.

147

68

STRADDLE JUMP—
used for shallow entry from a bank not more than one metre high.

Entry is made with the legs apart, body leaning forward at about 40 degrees to the vertical, arms extended sideways, slightly forwards and elbows bent a little. As soon as the water reaches waist level the legs will be closed vigorously and the hands pressed downwards. As a result RESCUER'S head should not submerge.

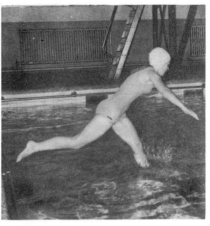

148

COMPACT JUMP—
used for entry from a height.

As RESCUER hits the water she will breathe out through her nose. Speed of descent through the water will be reduced by spreading the arms and kicking.

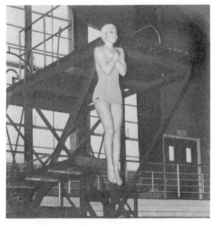

149

An alternative method of entering the water from a height.

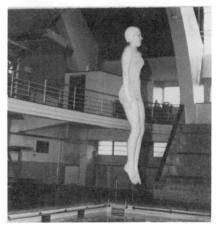

69   150

DEFENSIVE METHODS

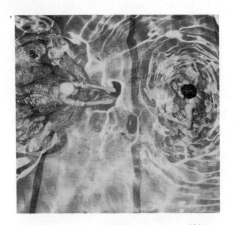

NOTE: All the defensive movements shown are for training purposes only. When making an actual rescue SUBJECT should always be approached from behind.

REVERSE.

RESCUER is approaching SUBJECT with a fast breast stroke.

151

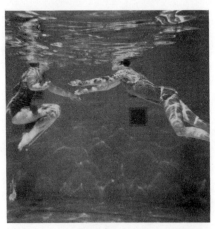

SUBJECT has suddenly lunged forward in an attempt to grasp RESCUER who is "braking" by extending her arms on either side, dropping her body and balling up in readiness to escape in the opposite direction.

152

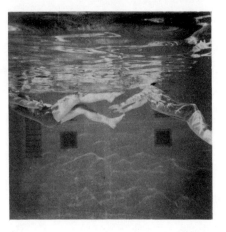

RESCUER is moving in the opposite direction using a back crawl kick and sculling strongly with her hands. At a safe distance, RESCUER will swim around SUBJECT in a large semi-circle, approach from behind and tow her back to the bank.

153

72

SINGLE LEG BLOCK

SUBJECT is reaching forward with her arms to grasp RESCUER who is braking and balling.

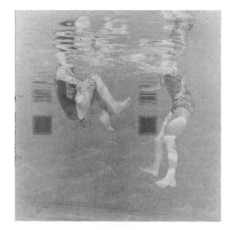

154

RESCUER has placed one foot on SUBJECT'S shoulder.

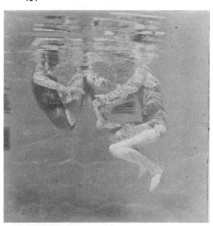

155

RESCUER has pushed herself away from SUBJECT. At a safe distance, RESCUER will swim around SUBJECT in a large semi-circle, approach from behind and tow her back to the bank.

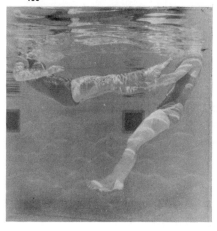

73   156

SINGLE LEG BLOCK COUNTER.

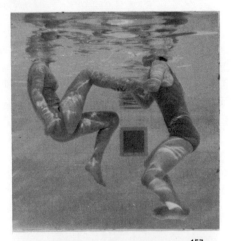

157

RESCUER has attempted a Single Leg Block, but her ankle has been grabbed by SUBJECT who is being jerked back towards RESCUER. RESCUER is taking advantage of this reaction by starting to depress the gripped leg as she bends it quickly to push SUBJECT under the water.

SUBJECT *must* hang on to RESCUER's ankle like a limpet throughout the push-pull.

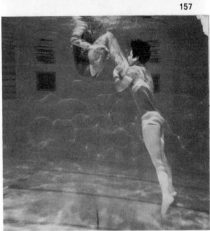

158

RESCUER immediately sculls forward with her hands and places her free foot on SUBJECT's other shoulder to push her down farther.

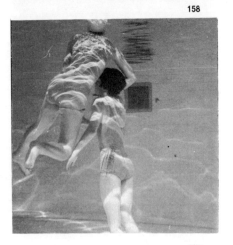

159

SUBJECT has released her hold in order to return to the surface for more air. RESCUER grasps SUBJECT by the chin as soon as her head rises to waist level to turn and raise her into a towing position.

DUCK AWAY.

SUBJECT has attempted to clutch RESCUER around the neck. RESCUER has quickly lowered her head and placed her hands on SUBJECT'S shoulders.

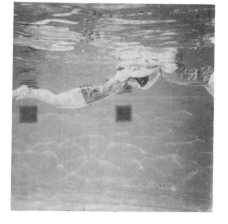

160

RESCUER is straightening her arms to push herself away from SUBJECT.

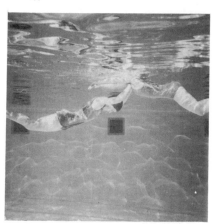

161

RESCUER is now clear of SUBJECT nd will surface out of range of urther clutches. At a safe distance, ESCUER will swim around SUBJECT in large semi-circle, approach from ehind and tow her back to the bank.

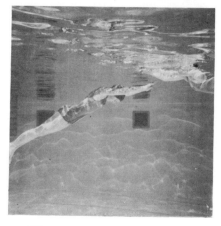

162

RELEASES

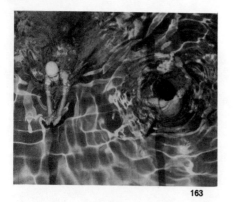

163

APPROACHING A DROWNING SUBJECT.

When making an actual rescue it is essential to avoid being grasped by the SUBJECT. The best method of achieving this is to approach the SUBJECT from behind.

RESCUER is swimming past SUBJECT at a distance of at least six feet.

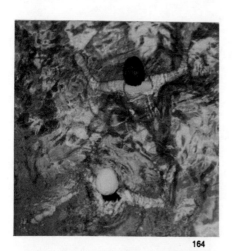

164

RESCUER has almost completed a large semi-circular turn. If SUBJECT is struggling violently RESCUER does not make contact until SUBJECT'S struggles have ceased indicating that she is exhausted.

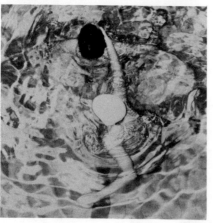

165

RESCUER has approached SUBJECT from behind and gripped her chin firmly with one hand prior to performing an extended tow. SUBJECT will be towed in a semi-circle back to the RESCUER'S original entry point.

RELEASE FROM FRONT CLUTCH ROUND BODY—
using Push Away Break.

RESCUER has placed her hands under SUBJECT's armpits and taken a deep breath.

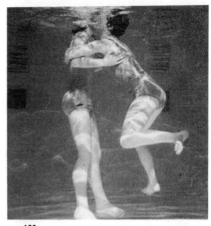

166

RESCUER has tucked her chin into her shoulder and submerged by forcing her elbows outwards and upwards against SUBJECT's arms.

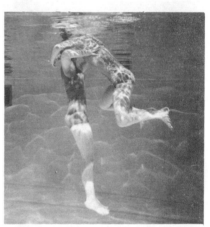

167

RESCUER has grasped SUBJECT's hips and started to spin her quickly around so that RESCUER will be behind SUBJECT.

NOTE: SUBJECT's clutch may be loose for the first few practices only. Thereafter SUBJECT must apply the strongest possible clutch and not release RESCUER until forced to do so. This is common to all the releases.

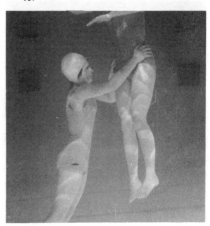

168

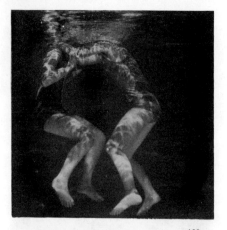

RELEASE FROM FRONT CLUTCH ROUND NECK—
using Push Away Break.

RESCUER has placed her hands under SUBJECT's elbows, taken a deep breath and tucked her chin in.

169

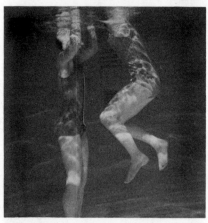

RESCUER has pushed SUBJECT's elbows upwards, impelling herself downwards.

170

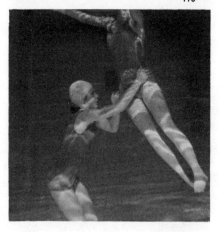

RESCUER has grasped SUBJECT's hips to spin her quickly so that SUBJECT's back will face RESCUER.

As soon as the hands have imparted the necessary spin, RESCUER will promptly swim back towards the surface in readiness to grasp SUBJECT's chin from behind and commence a tow.

171

RELEASE FROM WRIST GRIP—
using Pull Control.

SUBJECT has gripped RESCUER'S wrist.

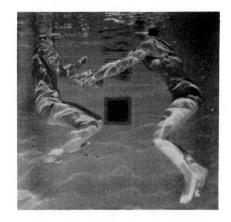

172

RESCUER has pulled SUBJECT towards herself with the gripped arm and passed her free arm around SUBJECT'S neck to grip the chin. At this point RESCUER is preparing to kick upwards to raise her shoulders above the surface of the water and pass farther behind SUBJECT.

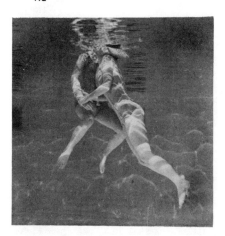

173

As RESCUER descends from her upward kick she presses her forearm on SUBJECT'S shoulder to sink her and free the gripped wrist.

After completing the release SUBJECT is towed in a semicircle back to RESCUER'S point of entry.

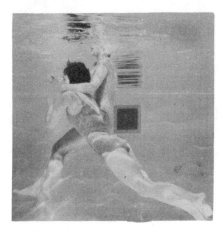

174

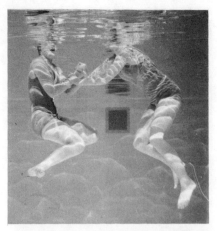

RELEASE FROM WRIST GRIP—
using Arm Pull Down.

RESCUER'S wrist has been gripped by SUBJECT with her thumbs underneath. RESCUER has clenched the fist of the gripped wrist and passed her free hand up between SUBJECT'S arms to grip the clenched fist.

175

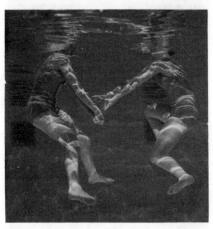

RESCUER has pulled her own clenched fist sharply downwards against SUBJECT'S thumbs to break the hold.

176

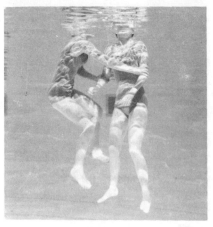

RESCUER has moved her hands quickly upwards to grasp SUBJECT just above her elbows. RESCUER is spinning SUBJECT into a towing position by pushing with one hand and pulling with the other.

177

RELEASE FROM WRIST GRIP—
using Arm Pull Up.

    RESCUER'S wrist has been gripped by SUBJECT with her thumbs on top of RESCUER'S wrist. RESCUER has passed her free hand down between SUBJECT'S arms to grip her own clenched fist.

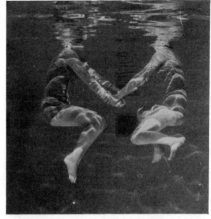

178

    RESCUER has pulled her own clenched fist sharply upwards against SUBJECT'S thumbs to break the hold.

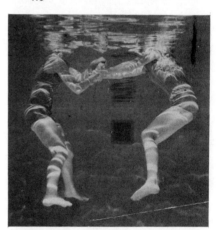

179

    RESCUER has moved her hands quickly forwards to grasp SUBJECT'S shoulders. RESCUER is spinning SUBJECT around with the intention of towing her.

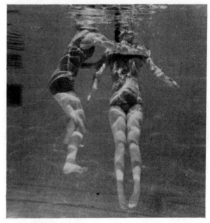

180

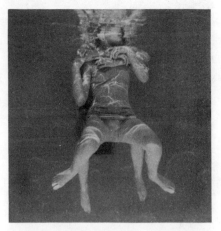

RELEASE FROM BACK CLUTCH ROUND NECK—
using Elbow Break.

RESCUER grasps SUBJECT'S uppermost arm at the wrist and elbow. RESCUER turns her head away from SUBJECT'S elbow and takes a deep breath.

181

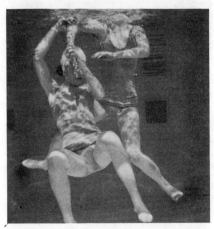

RESCUER pushes SUBJECT'S elbow up and pulls her wrist down. RESCUER submerges, passing under SUBJECT'S arm which is held at approximately a right angle and continuing the push on the elbow and the pull on the wrist.

182

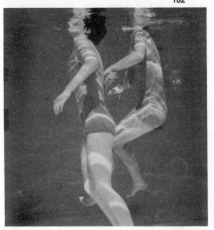

Using a rapid succession of powerful backstroke kicks RESCUER carries SUBJECT'S arm up behind her back.

N.B. To enable the reader to get a better view of the final action, both RESCUER and SUBJECT have turned clockwise through 90°.

183

RELEASE FROM BACK CLUTCH ROUND BODY—
using Joint Pressure Break.

RESCUER has grasped one of SUBJECT'S thumbs and the fingers of the other hand.

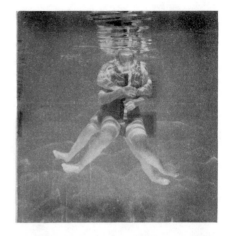

184

SUBJECT'S hold has been broken and RESCUER has spread SUBJECT'S arms wide to get clear.

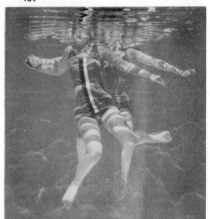

185

RESCUER has swum around behind SUBJECT and grasped her chin in readiness for towing.

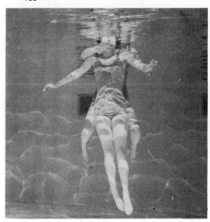

186

85

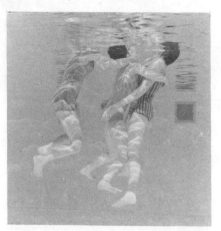

187

SEPARATION OF TWO SWIM-MERS LOCKED TOGETHER— with a body grip.

RESCUER has gripped the weaker SUBJECT'S chin firmly with both hands, fingers interlaced. RESCUER is bearing down with her forearms on the weaker SUBJECT'S shoulders to sink both of them.

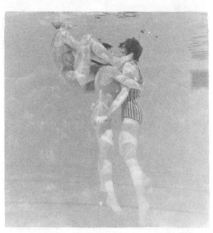

188

Having sunk both SUBJECTS, RESCUER is now able to place one foot on the stronger SUBJECT'S shoulder.

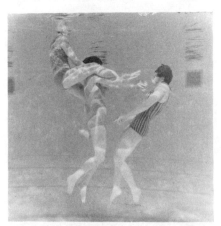

189

RESCUER has pushed with her foot and pulled with her hands to break the hold.

SEPARATION OF TWO SWIM-MERS LOCKED TOGETHER—
with a neck grip.

RESCUER has approached the weaker swimmer from behind, interlaced her fingers under SUBJECT'S chin and gripped it firmly. RESCUER'S forearms are bearing down on SUBJECT'S shoulders to sink her.

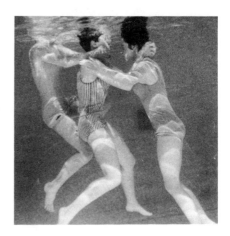

190

RESCUER has forced the weaker swimmer well down, making it easier to place her foot on the other swimmer's chest.

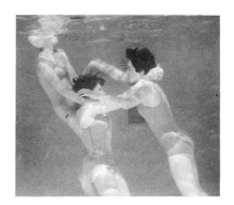

191

RESCUER is straightening her leg and pulling with her arms to break the hold.

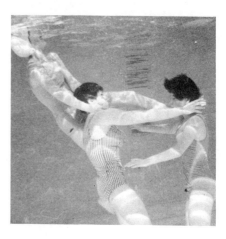

87

192

TOWS

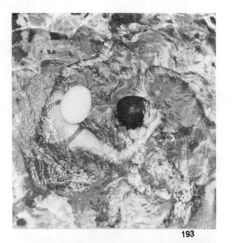

193

CHIN TOW.

RESCUER has approached SUBJECT from behind. Having extended her arm and gripped SUBJECT's chin RESCUER will pull SUBJECT's head quickly onto her shoulder, swing her hips forward and upward and commence the life saving back stroke kick using the free hand for sculling. Photographs 88-93 illustrate the fundamentals.

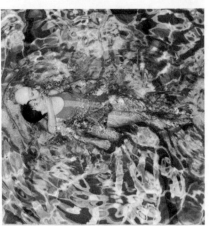

194

A rescuer should produce maximum power at the beginning of any tow in order to get both bodies moving and thus help to raise the SUBJECT's body into a reasonably horizontal position.

RESCUER has almost achieved the necessary speed of tow, but is still "revving" with rapid and powerful leg movements.

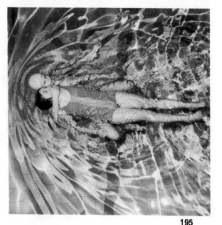

195

SUBJECT's face is turned toward RESCUER's face to enable RESCUER to press as much as possible of her forearm against SUBJECT's shoulder and chest thus improving control. RESCUER's free left hand is used to assist the tow by sculling.

[Continued on page 91.]

Shoulder Restraint

SUBJECT has started struggling and RESCUER has passed her free left hand under SUBJECT's armpit and gripped her left shoulder to obtain additional control. RESCUER continues with her life saving backstroke kick throughout the restraint.

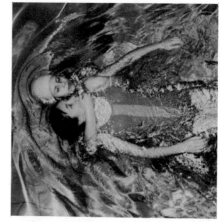

196

Breathing Restraint

SUBJECT has persisted with her struggling causing RESCUER to waste valuable energy in controlling her. RESCUER deters further struggling by pinching SUBJECT's nose between thumb and forefinger while the remainder of the same hand is pressed over SUBJECT's mouth completely stopping her breathing.

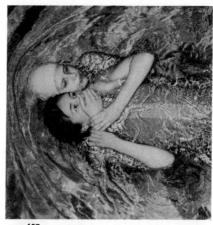

197

SUBJECT's immediate reaction is to pull RESCUER's arm down onto her chest and hold it there. RESCUER's free left hand can now be used to assist the tow by sculling again. Throughout the action RESCUER has maintained her life saving backstroke kick. The position shown may be maintained for the remainder of the tow.

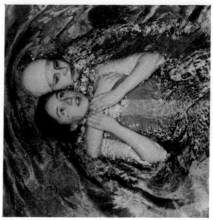

91

198

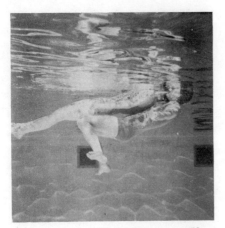

199

CHIN TOW—below surface view.

RESCUER'S legs have just begun the propulsive part of the life saving backstroke kick with both ankles turned outwards to provide a greater thrusting area to the water. RESCUER'S free hand is sculling and her body as horizontal as SUBJECT'S body will permit in order to reduce retardation

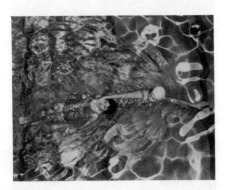

200

EXTENDED TOW— above surface view.

RESCUER is glancing at SUBJECT'S face to ensure it is above the surface of the water.

Photograph 96 gives fundamenta points of technique.

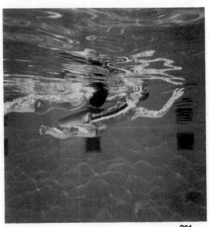

201

EXTENDED TOW— below surface view.

RESCUER'S body is as level as SUBJECT'S body will permit in order to minimise retardation.

CROSS CHEST TOW—
above surface view.

RESCUER'S towing arm is bent at approximately a right angle to avoid the possibility of the forearm bearing against SUBJECT's throat.

Photograph 94 gives fundamental points of technique.

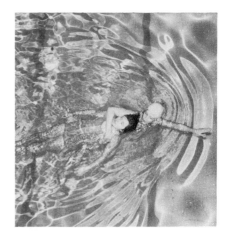

202

CROSS CHEST TOW—
below surface view.

SUBJECT'S back is held firmly against the side of RESCUER's chest. RESCUER's hips and legs are as horizontal as SUBJECT's bottom will permit in order to reduce retardation.

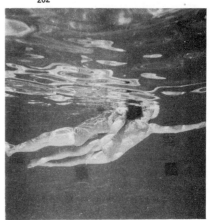

203

CROSS CHEST TOW—
with restraint—above surface view.

RESCUER has obtained greater control of SUBJECT by gripping her shoulder firmly with the free hand. RESCUER has turned onto her back and is using the life saving back-stroke kick.

After SUBJECT's struggles cease, RESCUER will revert to the technique illustrated in photographs 202 and 203.

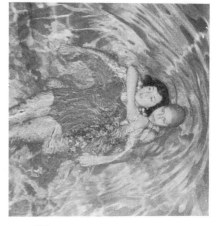

204

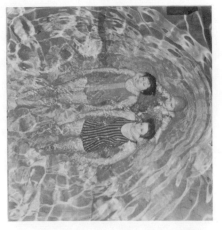

DOUBLE RESCUE TOW—
by the chin with extended arms.

A tow for advanced life savers requiring power and stamina.

Photograph 98 gives fundamental points of technique.

205

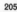

DOUBLE RESCUE TOW—
by the chin with bent arms.

206

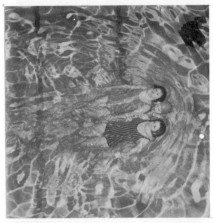

DOUBLE RESCUE TOW—
by the hair with extended arms.

The easiest of the three variation shown—provided SUBJECTS have sufficient hair to grasp. Because RESCUER is farther away from SUBJECTS' bodies she can raise her own body into a flatter position, thu reducing her own retardation and increasing her towing speed.

207

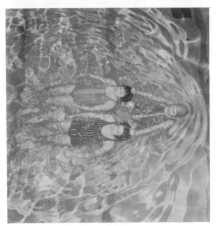

LANDINGS

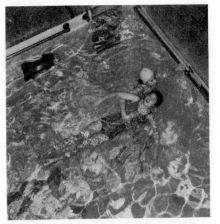

LANDING A RESCUED SUBJECT
—from deep water—preliminary movements.

When RESCUER is approximately three feet from the bank at the completion of a tow, one hand is placed just below SUBJECT'S sternum and the other hand grasps the rail.

208

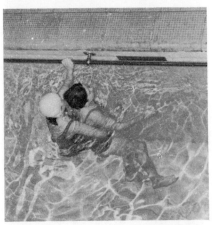

RESCUER holds SUBJECT firmly against her right front side as she turns to face the bank.

209

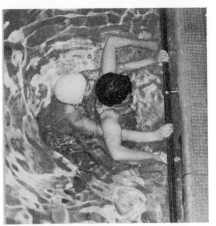

As soon as RESCUER passes her right hand under SUBJECT'S right armpit to grip the rail, she releases her left hand hold and quickly passes that hand under SUBJECT'S left armpit to grip the bar again. RESCUER is shown in the "support position".

210

96

SUBJECT'S hand and wrist are placed on the bank.

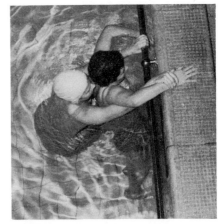

211

While holding SUBJECT'S right hand firmly on the bank, RESCUER grasps SUBJECT'S left hand and places it on top of SUBJECT'S other hand.

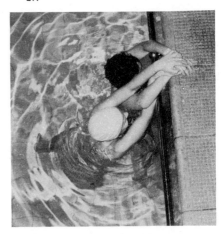

212

Maintaining a firm vertical pressure on both SUBJECT'S hands, RESCUER moves slightly to the right and places her free hand on the bank in readiness to leave the water.

[This concludes the preliminary movements which are used for both the Crossed Arm and Straight Arm methods of landing.]

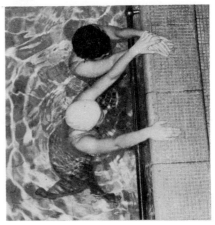

213

97

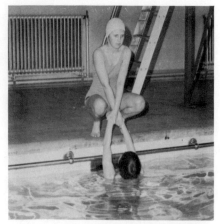

LANDING A RESCUED SUBJECT
—from deep water—using Crossed Arm Method.

As RESCUER leaves the water she maintains a strong pressure on both SUBJECT's hands with her left hand. RESCUER pivots around her vertical left arm until she faces SUBJECT. RESCUER's free right hand grasps SUBJECT's right wrist, the left hand then grasps SUBJECT's left wrist. RESCUER, her wrists crossed is now ready for the lift.

214

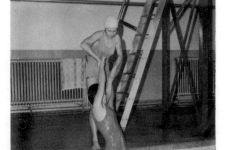

RESCUER, keeping SUBJECT's face above the water, raises and lowers her a few times to obtain impetus. In making the full lift RESCUER's arms are uncrossed thus turning SUBJECT's back to the bank.

To minimise the possibility of back injury, RESCUER should hollow her back slightly and make her leg muscles provide practically all the lifting power.

215

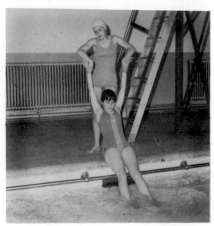

At the instant that the maximum height of lift is achieved, RESCUER takes two very quick steps backwards as she pulls, to ensure that SUBJECT will achieve a secure sitting position on the bank.

216

LANDING A RESCUED SUBJECT
—from deep water—using Straight Arm Method.

Placing SUBJECT's hands on the bank and leaving the water have already been described [photographs 211-214.]

RESCUER's arms are not crossed. SUBJECT will be raised (water at waist level) and lowered (water *below* face level) a few times to gain impetus.

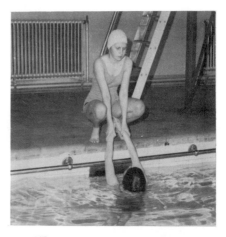

217

Having extended her legs to obtain the full lift, RESCUER instantly moves two steps backwards to land the upper part of the SUBJECT's body on the bank. SUBJECT—assumed to be unconscious—must *not* bend her arms to assist RESCUER's lift.

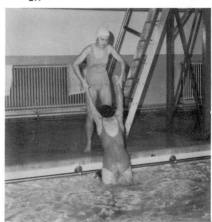

218

RESCUER holds SUBJECT firmly in position with one hand on her back while using the other hand to lift SUBJECT's legs onto the bank.

NOTE: This technique requires less lifting effort than the Crossed Arm Method but needs more time for its completion.

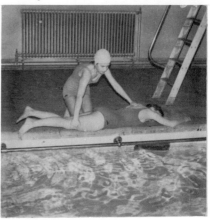

219

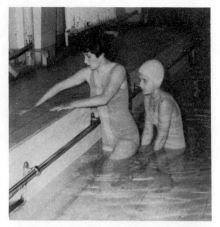

LANDING A RESCUED SUBJECT
—from shallow water—using Stirrup Method.

RESCUER standing behind SUBJECT instructs her to "place both hands on the bank and raise your left foot". SUBJECT complies with the instructions while RESCUER interlaces her fingers.

220

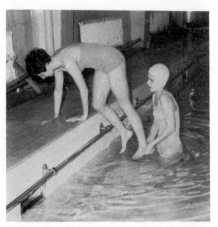

RESCUER supports SUBJECT's foot with her interlaced fingers, gripping the foot firmly. RESCUER instructs SUBJECT to "straighten your leg and push up with your arms". RESCUER then straightens her own knees and further assists the lift by bending her arms.

221

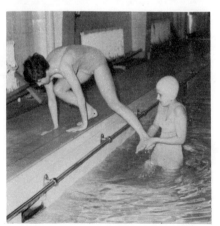

SUBJECT lands.

RESCUER should endeavour to keep her back as vertical as possible throughout the landing and provide most of the lifting power with her legs.

222

EXPIRED AIR RESUSCITATION
IN WATER

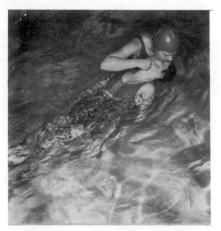

EXPIRED AIR RESUSCITATION
—Standing in Shallow Water.

RESCUER is simulating the mouth-to-nose technique with SUBJECT'S neck extended and exhaling audibly beyond her far cheek. RESCUER is walking sideways towards the bank as quickly as possible. RESCUER'S other hand supports SUBJECT'S trunk either between her shoulder blades or under her far armpit.

223

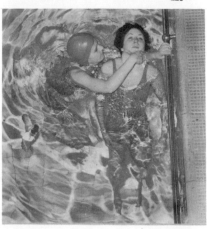

EXPIRED AIR RESUSCITATION
—Supported in Deep Water.

RESCUER grasps the handrail and supports SUBJECT'S neck on her arm. RESCUER'S other hand grasps SUBJECT'S jaw, pushing upwards towards the top of SUBJECT'S head to close her mouth and extend the neck in readiness for mouth-to-nose resuscitation.

224

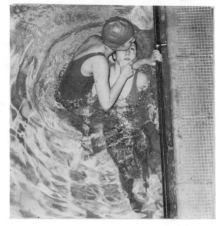

By pulling with the hand grasping the handrail and kicking rapidly with her legs, RESCUER rises over SUBJECT'S face to simulate expiration for mouth-to-nose resuscitation and exhales audibly.

225   102

EXPIRED AIR RESUSCITATION
—Swimming in Deep Water.

RESCUER is using the Chin Tow.

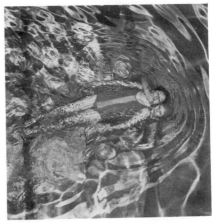

226

RESCUER has extended her arm and moved around to the other side of SUBJECT, adjusting her hand hold in readiness for mouth-to-nose resuscitation. RESCUER's free hand is placed at the back of SUBJECT's head. Throughout these manoeuvres RESCUER maintains as much speed as possible using the life saving backstroke kick

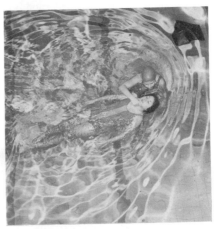

227

By kicking rapidly and powerfully upwards, RESCUER raises herself sufficiently to apply her mouth to SUBJECT's forehead and exhales audibly. RESCUER maintains as much speed as possible towards the bank throughout the action and must not submerge SUBJECT's face.

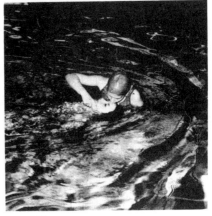

228

103

INDEX